I0426788

A crucial element has been missing
from the world of weight loss plans...
...until now

CHUBBY NO MORE
THE COMFORT CONNECTION

...linking weight loss programs with
lasting success through comfort

A GUIDEBOOK

THREE STEPS FOR BUILDING
THE POWER OF PERMANENCE
INTO ANY WEIGHT LOSS METHOD

By

Pamela Aye Simon, M.S, R.D., L.D

© 2003 by Pamela Aye Simon, M.S, R.D., L.D.
All rights reserved.

No part of this book may be reproduced, stored in a
retrieval system, or transmitted by any means, electronic,
mechanical, photocopying, recording, or otherwise, without
written permission from the author.

ISBN: 1-4107-4740-9 (e-book)
ISBN: 1-4107-4741-7 (Paperback)

This book is printed on acid free paper.

Cover design by Jenna and Pam Simon

1stBooks - rev. 6/10/03

DISCLAIMER

The ideas expressed in this writing are solely those of the author, and do not necessarily represent those of the profession of dietetics as a whole. The concepts presented are based on her professional practice as a registered dietitian and on her personal experience.

The steps and exercises which are explained in this book are not intended to be used as a substitute for medical or psychiatric treatment. In no way should these practices replace care required by physicians or counselors. Prescribed medications should not be changed without direct orders from the prescribing physician.

The book offers guidelines, which may help the reader achieve improved body confidence. These steps do hold the potential of enhancing self esteem, and therefore may contribute to progress made with other self-improvement programs or medical treatment plans.

DEDICATION

These words are dedicated...

to my beautiful daughter and wisest teacher, Jenna Wind Simon, who has an amazing ability to feel the joy and see the hope in all situations,

to my husband Stanton, whose love is always present,

to my mom, my hero, who is a living example of the concepts in this book,

to my dad, who taught me to attempt the impossible,

to my brother, who courageously seeks answers to the hardest questions,

and to Dr. Monica, who has given me the chance to walk above my darkness.

"With professional expertise and personal knowledge, Pam Aye Simon offers an impressive new vision for lasting weight loss. If you are tired of the endless array of weight loss programs promising results which never seem to last, here is a solid way to ADD ON to your chosen plan. This inclusive approach can complement individual efforts and all weight loss programs by supplying an often overlooked but crucial key to successful and permanent results. *The Comfort Connection should be the companion book for all individuals involved in the weight loss process.*"

Linda O'Toole, M.S., R.D.

Imagine yourself light enough
to fly up to the stars.
If this challenges you,
then we will surround you with comfort.
When your comfort is deep enough
you will find the wings to fly.

(pas)

✕

ACKNOWLEDGEMENTS

I would like to thank the many people who have been there for me over time, especially:
Art Dobbins, for watching over us,
My dear friends, Jane Bobowicz, Linda O'Toole, Cathy Buffa, Ellen Plank, Joe Shearin and Gay, Maureen, Kathy, who all put up with my lagging communication skills,
George at Cyber Exchange, who provided my laptop,
The staff at Mail Boxes Etc., for the office support,
Mike and his employees at Chuckie Cheese's, for keeping my daughter busy while I worked,
Eleanor Betz, Mary Castellanos, Dr. Dowling, Ms. Barry, Dr. Tangney, Dr. Bowen, Dr. Prewitt, Dr. Schmeisser, Dr. Kamath, Maria Sapuntzakus, who made a difference in my professional path,
The Arlington Heights Chamber of Commerce and PWC,
Barb Jakomin at Village Profile, for putting me on the map,
Mindy & Jim Elgas for the Almanac support,
Ron at Quinlin and Fabish, for emergency horn repair,
And finally, the ladies of Baroque Babes, and all my musician friends who keep me playing.

TABLE OF CONTENTS

INTRODUCTION

A SALUTE TO THE WEIGHT WARRIORS

How do you feel about your body image right now? Do you carry around negative feelings about your weight,
your fitness level, or your eating habits?

If you have moments in your day when you feel guilty about what you eat, what you weigh, or how you look, this book is for you. If you are too tired to try another exercise class, read on. Even if you refuse to alter your eating plan, or feel like you just found the perfect diet, there is something here for you.

But first, a tribute is in order, and long overdue.

For all of you who have struggled with weight loss plans,
I salute you and your fighting spirit. *You are remarkable.*

And yet...

...you are rarely given credit for the battles you fight. More often than not, you are blamed for not fighting hard enough.

You seem to bounce back.

If one weight loss method doesn't work, you rarely give up for long. You get the strength to try another.

Your self-esteem suffers terribly, yet much of your pain is kept hidden. You don't blame others for the struggle.

You tend to place all the blame on yourself.

You may have years of great success and the highest hope that the battle has been won. But just when you think you can relax, the weight battle begins again.

This book is a salute to you. You are the embodiment of the spirits of hope, persistence and courage.
You are a hero.

In this book, I offer you a different path...one which soothes and comforts. This path provides a connection between you and the body image of your dreams. The element that has been missing from your efforts is the very thing you thought you couldn't have - increased feelings of deep comfort to replace the pain and guilt.

Enough with the guilt.
Enough with the pain.

Right now, you need comfort.
Then you can get down to the business of weight loss.

CHAPTER ONE

I'M DIETING AS FAST AS I CAN

Losing weight can be a challenge for just about anyone. Maintaining weight loss for more than two years seems to baffle the best of us (dieters and health professionals alike).

We all want to blame someone or something! But the failure of maintaining weight loss should NEVER be blamed on the individual. And yet, many times, I have seen the guilt and blame directed at him or her by family, friends, health care professionals.

We need a much more healing approach.

We need to build, not blame. The fault lies not with the individual, the program nor the professional. *In fact, I believe that the inability to achieve and/or maintain weight loss has very little to do with what you eat.*

In the pages of this book, you will learn how one simple addition to your existing efforts can connect you to a more lasting change.

That is what it did for me...

Just like you, I am a survivor. I have lived through more weight loss diets, pills and exercise routines than I can remember. I have survived addictive and strange eating behaviors and consuming preoccupation with my weight...but not anymore.

I am also a registered dietitian with years of experience in the weight loss counseling field.

Today, when one of my clients says:

"Give me a diet, I have to lose weight," I hesitate.

I just don't have the heart to add any more guilt to the shoulders of someone who may still be carrying feelings of failure from past diets.

My experience tells me that the diet by itself just won't work. Pounds might come off, but they may as easily come back.

Within 2 years, the weight seems to be regained and feelings of failure and guilt increase. This failure isn't the fault of the individual or of the weight loss program.

Something has definitely been missing.

For all of the suffering, hard work and progress—including various diet plans, fitness programs, surgical procedures and diet pills, weight change just doesn't seem to last.

We have all tried to find the reason, but we have had our hands full! From the individuals who try to lose weight, to the professionals searching for new strategies to help their clients, we have all been very busy.

It has been difficult to find the time and space to stand back and see the whole picture.

As a result, most of our programs address the physical change desired, but we have not addressed the vital process of mental and emotional adjustment to the change. This aspect could very well be big enough to block long-term, successful weight loss.

*There should be as much emphasis on changing the **inside** of the individual so that he or she can* prepare for, and become comfortable with, the good body changes.

It is really the whole person who needs attention—*the body, the mind and the spirit.*

In other words, your emotional comfort should grow bigger as you get smaller.

CHAPTER TWO

ALL ABOUT ME, ME, ME, AND YOU

A very crucial part of the process has been missing. In the world of weight loss programs, the addition of this part could change the long-term results completely.

I believe this because I found out the hard way. It took many years. But today I can honestly say that I am able to live without thoughts of food and body weight, and with no feelings of guilt. This is pretty amazing, because I have probably been dieting longer than many of you have been alive.

My first dieting experience was "The Grapefruit and Cottage Cheese Diet." (I went on this one with my dad.) The last was the "Eat a Box of Cookies-a-Day Diet." (This one was my very own invention—but it worked as well as any other.)

There were many other weight loss diets in between. The "Eat only Vegetables Diet" and the "Eat 10 Snacks-a-Day (but no meals) Diet" were two of the most memorable. Then there were all the exercise plans, like the "Yoga Stretch (between meals of lettuce) Program," and the "Run-Around-the-Yard Plan" (my mom's idea). And guess what? I did lose weight...

...again, and again, and again.

And I gained back the lost weight...

...again, and again, and again.

Let's face it. It doesn't take a complete genius to realize that something wasn't working. Sure, I could lose weight. But I kept finding it again - along with lots of guilt. (I wonder if guilt attached to a pound of body weight results in a pound that weighs twice as much? That could explain a lot!)

So - I kept doing the same thing over and over and expecting different results.

This miserable cycle of...

diet>>>weight-loss>>>whoops!>>>weight gain>>>diet

...was...what?...not working?

It took me a long time to get this one.

But finally after the exhausting years of dieting and exercise activities, culminating in the "Eat All the Cookies You Want Diet," the light went on. I was missing something.

There was something missing from my various weight loss efforts.

And I thought I knew what it was.

There will always be another eating plan, pill, or exercise program which promises to be more successful for weight loss than all the others.

There will always be one that looks different, one that promises to hold the secret. I was not falling for it this time!

I wanted to stop this craziness. I felt like a jilted lover. The relationship I had with my body image and diets was highly dysfunctional. It was also robbing me of my self worth...

...one calorie at a time.

I wanted to live life.

I was weary of driving down the street and noticing the advertisements for food and restaurants...

...instead of looking up at the trees and sky.

I was tired of counting calories.

I longed to count the stars instead...

I longed for a bigger life...

CHAPTER THREE

BUY A NEW BATHING SUIT

Maybe I simply wasn't ready for the changes to happen. I hadn't prepared the *emotional* me for the *physical* changes. No one told me I needed to think of this, but now it made sense. Becoming a thinner person wasn't totally comfortable for me because I wasn't used to it. My internal body mold was too big now for the thinner, physical me.

I hadn't been aware of this feeling before. Yet I knew the feeling was not new. It had just been hiding below the surface of my awareness.

I FELT STANGE. I felt like I lost weight but forgot to buy a new bathing suit!

I felt a draft! I felt exposed!

To put it another way, I felt like cookie dough that is too small for the cookie cutter...too much space. There was a space inside me that needed to be filled.

I felt mentally/emotionally overweight even though I was physically thinner.

Although I loved being the thinner person, there was a part of me that wanted to bring back the *overweight-me.* Deep down, I felt safer when my body size stayed the same. The *overweight-me* was someone I had known a long time. *She* wouldn't put me in danger. *She* was a friend.

Of course I wanted to be thinner! I just wasn't sure I wanted to hang out with the new *thinner-body- me.* This *thinner-body-me* was a stranger. She did not make me feel warm and fuzzy.

Sure, I was now living in her body, but I didn't feel as safe as before. She was unfamiliar and threatening. I wasn't sure I was prepared for what this thinner person would make me do.

What if she signed me up for power yoga, or made me give up chocolate, or wanted to "dress for success" everyday...or worse?

Was I ready for all this?

Not quite, but I knew what I had to do.

Before diets, pills, exercise programs, stomach surgery, etc. can help in attaining permanent weight loss, the individual has to feel deeply comfortable about being a thinner person.

I believe that the major reason for weight-loss failure over time has everything to do with an individual's state of readiness for living in a thinner body.

For me, I thought I wanted, more than anything, to look better and feel better. But on some level, I still saw myself as the out-of-shape me, the person who believed it when someone told her that she would "get fat just like Daddy." Over the years, I got a lot of practice with this feeling. It was safe and familiar. I was used to it...like a worn sweat suit, or an old shoe. And unless I could change my emotional comfort level to include a better-body me, weight loss wouldn't feel OK.

I had to get ready for success.

Just as in any construction project, the foundation MUST be in place for the rest of the building to remain stable. A permanent weight change requires foundational work as well.

The weight loss process does not automatically include a plan for emotional adjustment—you have to take care of this.

Just because you may have wanted to be thinner for a long time, don't assume you will naturally feel wonderful when it happens.

FEELING COMFORTABLE with the changes that come with weight loss SUCCESS is not automatic - it takes practice.

In the chapters that follow, you will learn how to add this crucial (but simple) method to your existing lifestyle with only 5-10 minutes a day of delightful mental exercises. This method teaches how to become emotionally ready for success in weight management, so that you finally stop attracting the weight you lost. Changes in your body require changes in your mind and heart if they are to last.

This is not a complicated process. But the results are amazing.

CHAPTER FOUR/STEP ONE

LOSE THE GUILT

Weight loss plans and guilt feelings are supposed to go together—right? And these guilt feelings are really good motivators, right?

NO

In fact, I believe that the exact opposite is true. You cannot live in guilt and have lasting successful weight loss at the same time. In order to lay the foundation for that success you have to see and feel yourself as a very strong, courageous and amazing person. Guilt doesn't serve a purpose.

STOP FEELING GUILTY about weight and food.*

The first step in the process of growing comfortable with success is this: shake off the guilt. You have control over this. Guilt feelings are just a habit, and as silly as it sounds, you have to practice living without them.

For me, I was afraid that if I didn't spend at least some time blaming myself for unrestricted eating behaviors, I would lose control completely.

---

* This is not to be confused with true, specific guilt, associated with an action or event. In this case, the person needs to make amends as appropriate.

That didn't happen. In fact, I gained more control, and felt much better.

Losing the guilt can certainly help you feel better about yourself, and this will increase your comfort level with success. Guilt about eating and weight only serves to add pounds in the long run.

Don't ever dwell on what you should have done, or didn't do in situations regarding eating or exercise (like, "I shouldn't have eaten..." Or "I should be going to the health club...") STOP. You do not deserve to be beaten up by guilt. It serves no purpose.

Sure, at first, guilt and fear may help to get you started. But I have seen that, in the long run, it hinders positive results, and may do more to rob you of weight loss success than almost any other influence.

You have to get rid of it, and still feel comfortable.

But how do you get rid of guilt in a simple way?

It just takes practice.

The exercise that worked for me is the one I describe here, and encourage you to try. You may develop variations of this that suit your style. But remember that you are undoing years of habitual guilt feelings. To stop the guilt habit you need two things: repetition and written words. This combination has a powerful effect.

Practice for 2 minutes each day, with the following exercise:

With paper and pen, write the words "I am free of guilt about my weight/eating/exercise habits today," (or you your own wording for the same message) for 1 minute each morning and I minute each evening. I know this sounds silly. I laughed at the idea until I tried it. But it worked. It took a few days of feeling silly and going through the motions. But the words you write will eventually reach your feelings.

You will actually feel energized as guilt drops

away. You are now clearing the way for the

next step.

CHAPTER FIVE/STEP TWO

CREATING NEW PAY-OFFS

Please read this chapter with an open mind and an open heart. This step requires awareness of a vital part of your emotional self. Adjustment to weight change may be more complete when this is addressed.

I believe that all of us have a part inside of us which sometimes feels like a scared child. This is the piece of us that wants to stay in the same, safe place. It is a quiet voice in our hearts that seeks to protect us from emotional annihilation. For some of us, the voice is too soft to hear. Others are well aware of its sound. Either way, its influence seems to be quite powerful.

For example, there are some aspects to being over weight that may help increase feelings of safety and comfort. Recognizing this fact and changing it has been crucial in helping me and others connect to permanent weight loss.

Think about it - you have probably lived with your overweight-self for a while. It is familiar and it seems safe. And, believe it or not, there are some positive pay-offs for remaining this way. One obvious pay-off is that you can keep things the same, which offers a certain level of comfort. You don't have to change your activities, eating habits, or exercise routine...the list goes on. These pay-offs are hard to give up, because they comfort you and protect you from the unknown. Some aren't even quite on the conscious level. And guess what - we all have these! This brings us to the next step.

You need to identify some of these pay-offs. You do not need to analyze deeply or take very long to do this. You don't need to come up with all of the details. These comfort areas exist, and should be recognized. What makes you want to stay in the overweight zone?

For me, it was just plain scary to think of walking anywhere and having people notice me. I wanted to feel invisible.

And as long as I felt like I didn't look very good, I figured no one would look my way. Also, I didn't worry about being well-dressed, wearing a bikini, and so on.

Here are some examples of pay-offs you may identify:

- You don't have to worry about being in style

- You have a reason to stay in the house

- You don't have to go swimming with...

And so on. Do this once.

Then move on to the second part of this step.

This part is very important. Imagine that you are the thin person you long to be. What are some of the wonderful ways you will feel the benefits of being thinner?

You need to create new, comfortable and soothing pay-offs for the thinner person you are becoming. Again, this takes practice. Feelings of comfort are key.

If you haven't spent much time in your life as a thin person, practice this step diligently. You are helping that little scared kid inside you feel more secure with changes that occur in your body weight.

You have to picture some rewards you may experience as a thinner person that are comforting, soothing and wonderful - new comfort pay-offs.

Some examples would be:

I hear my daughter whisper in my ear that I look beautiful

I have more energy when I wake up in the morning

I try on jeans that are 2 sizes smaller, and they fit!

I can wear PJs all day and still feel thin, and so on.

Now for the exercise which puts this step into action:

Write this down with pen and paper:

Imagine some of the rewards you might experience when you have a better body. Are some of these new pay-offs scary or threatening? Cross these out. Are some of the pay-offs really comforting to think about? Write these down again. Be totally aware of how you feel when you imagine the pay-offs.

Do this for 1 minute each morning and one minute in the evening. You need to be able to come up with at least five better-body pay-offs that feel really good. Keep doing this daily.

CHAPTER SIX/ STEP THREE

PAINT A NEW PICTURE

This is a great step. It takes the old phrase: "you are what you eat," and expands it to the more meaningful and delightful words: "you are what you think (feel, believe, etc)." The successful outcome of your weight loss plan depends mainly upon the way you think about yourself. If you have lots of negative images of yourself and your weight, these images need to be changed. They are old pictures, and need to be replaced with new ones. You need to become emotionally comfortable with your mental pictures of the new you.

The great news is this: With practice, these new images can become part of you, and will then affect how you respond to your desire to change.

In other words, the more you practice changing your thoughts of yourself to those that paint a better picture of the person you can become, the better chance you have of losing weight and keeping it off - and with a lot more comfort.

When I first thought of this step, I was doubtful of its effectiveness. I spent too long in graduate school and the world of nutrition research to ever trust any method that wasn't backed up by numerous documented reports.

But personally speaking, I needed a little speck of hope.

That speck of hope is all it took.

And that is all you need.

The next step in the comfort process can change you completely.

Please practice this step for 2 minutes in the morning and two minutes in the evening.

With pen and paper, record the following:

Imagine that you are the thinner person you desire to be. Describe yourself in positive ways as if it were happening in the present, like "I am thin and confident..." Imagine what you are wearing, doing, saying, feeling, thinking, etc. Imagine in color.

Your feelings are especially important, as are all the details you can picture. This may seem ridiculous at first. Don't let that stop you. Your mental picture of the physical person you want to be may feel unrealistic, but shouldn't seem impossible. It may feel slightly foreign, but shouldn't create stress.

With practice, the best image for you will become clear.

Do not give up on the practice of this step for anything. You may have days, hours, moments when it seems like nonsense. Practice anyway. The negativity will pass. You may not have the time to put anything in writing. If that is the case, close your eyes and think this step. Do this step each day, no matter what.

Continue to hold the image of who you want to be in your mind's eye. As you spend time daily with this mental picture, you will feel much more comfortable with the new you.

Never give this up.

Weight loss success will naturally follow. Other great changes may happen. You may experience much greater ease in following your chosen weight loss plan, fitness program, etc. You may want to take a break from defined eating plans. You may even find you have an inherent desire to make healthier choices.

Why?

Your new emotional comfort level is now connecting you to the dreams you once thought impossible. And this is only the beginning...

CHAPTER SEVEN

PUTTING IT TOGETHER

Finally, let's put all the steps to the Comfort Connection Method together:

1. LOSE THE GUILT

Practice for 2 minutes each day:

Write the words "I am free of guilt about my weight/eating/exercise habits today," (or you your own wording for the same message) for 1 minute each morning and I minute each evening. The words you write will eventually reach your feelings.

2. <u>CREATE NEW PAY-OFFS</u>

Practice for 2 minutes twice a day:

Write *some of the rewards you might experience when you have a better body.*

Are some of these new pay-offs scary or threatening? Cross these out. Are some of the pay-offs really comforting to think about? Write these down again.

Be totally aware of how you feel when you imagine the pay-offs. You need to be able to come up with at least five better-body pay-offs that feel really good.

3. <u>PAINT A BETTER PICTURE</u>

Practice this step for 2 minutes twice a day:

Record the following: imagine that you are the thinner person you desire to be.

Describe yourself in detailed, positive ways, as if it were happening in the present (like "I am at a party at my house, wearing a black dress, and feeling thin and confident...").
Imagine what you are wearing, doing, saying, feeling, thinking, etc. Imagine in color Your feelings are especially important, as are all the details you can picture. Come up with as many different scenarios as you can. With

practice, the best image for you will become

clear.

In conclusion: your thoughts and written words

are treasures. Keep them safe from the eyes and

ears of anyone who may not understand. Don't allow

any outside opinions to minimize or criticize your

work.

You may not always be able to practice the steps

in a quiet place with a pen and paper. That doesn't

matter. Take mental quiet time and do the

exercises in your imagination.

Your goal is to become familiar and comfortable

with an image of yourself as successful in

permanent weight loss. You may use variations of the above steps, or add strategies of your own creation.

Finally, the process of developing the comfort connection with successful weight loss is simple, but not easy. Daily practice, repetition, and your own written words give power to your efforts, and bring success closer to you.

Throughout the process, keep in mind that no one is just like you. Your thoughts and feelings are yours alone…fragile, delicate and precious. Hold them very close to you. Then relax.

Because, the tiniest amount of self-belief can change everything

A speck of hope is all it takes...

I stared into the child's eyes

And was surprised to see

The wisdom of the heavens

Waiting there for me.

(PAS)

CHAPTER EIGHT

Q AND A

Q.

Do I have to practice this method for the rest of my life for lasting results?

A.

Yes and no. With daily practice, the positive body image you have created will take hold on a deeper level. The process becomes part of who you are. Over time, the positive images automatically replace negative ones.

But no matter what, you need to do the exercises everyday, even when things are going great, and especially after you have lost the desired amount of weight.

Q.

How long do I have to practice before the positive images become automatic?

A.

That depends on how severe your negative body imagery has become. On average, at the end of 3 months of daily practice, the process should be integrated into your thoughts. It should seem easier to do.

Q.

What should my eating plan be while I am learning all of this?

A.

You can follow any healthy food plan of your choice. But you need to relax about eating, and to not feel guilty about your eating during this time.

Q.

What if I feel just too silly imagining myself as thin?

A.

Take baby steps. The first week, imagine yourself 3 pounds thinner, then 5, 7, and so on. It will work.

The big question is: How much do you want it? If you are not ready yet, wait until you can't stand feeling yukky about the way you look, feel, etc. You will know when the time is right.

Q.

Why do some people have a lot less trouble staying thin than other people?

A.

I am not sure we really know the total answer to that question. It may be a combination of factors, like genetics, eating habits metabolic rate, etc. For most of us, however, I believe we can still change our weight loss success by working with body image.

In my family, my grandmother, great grandmother, and great grandfather were obese. My dad was over weight. If I can fight a pattern like this, so can you!

Q.

Can't you just tell me specifically how many calories I need to lose weight, and then plan meals for me? Isn't that what a dietitian does? I just need you to tell me what to do.

A.

Many dietitians will do this for you. A calorie-controlled eating plan is one way, if you feel a need for that. Make sure you secure the services of a **Registered Dietitian**. She or he would be the most qualified. Keep in mind there are many options available.

But, along with any food plan, using the Comfort Connection Method can help ease the pain of the process. From my experience, the diet and method used together could greatly enhance your chances

of achieving and maintaining weight loss.

Q.

What about the supplements that claim to burn

fat or carbohydrates? Couldn't that help also?

A.

If there were a pill which offered a safe and

permanent solution to weight loss, we would ALL be

taking it, wouldn't we? I sure would! As a

professional registered dietitian, I can't

recommend these products for my clients, simply

because research evidence on efficacy and

effectiveness is not yet complete.

It is possible that any number of products have potential in the weight loss area. At the present time, however, I believe the most solid solution to permanent weight loss is a balanced diet (ALL foods included) and positive body image work.

Q.

Is it OK to just accept myself as a heavy person, and stop trying to be the thin person I am not?

A.

What a great question! Yes. It is time for all of us to accept ourselves for what we are today. I should have put that factor in the chapter on losing the guilt.

The great thing about accepting the present you, is that once you do this, you can feel and see more clearly whether you actually WANT to lose weight.

Of course, I have a professional obligation to advise weight loss for anyone who is moderately overweight, for health reasons alone.

Q.

You say in the book to ease up on eating restrictions while first learning the comfort connection. I am a binger. If I ease up, there is no telling how much I will eat. It is scary.

A.

If the eating really scares you, the first action to be taken is to consult with an eating disorder specialist. A true eating disorder can be dangerous, and may have brain chemistry abnormalities. There are some great medications that can provide substantial help once an eating disorder diagnosis is made.

Otherwise, it seems that most people who have been restricting food intake do experience feelings of anger at being deprived of the amounts of favorite foods desired. These feelings can build frustration levels to the point where eating control gives way to saying "the hell with this," and follow it by binging behavior.

There actually is a solution to this kind of binging. This solution may sound like the exact opposite of what you think you should do, but it worked for me...really worked.

Here it is: for the next 2 weeks, have no restrictions on your eating. Eat anything you want, at any time you want, in any quantity you wish.*

You won't believe what happens next.

You will actually grow tired of the foods you have been longing for, and you will have no feelings of deprivation. It will feel comfortable. You also will have no reason to binge anymore.

During this time, allow yourself to eat cake for dinner or ice cream for lunch. Please do not force yourself to eat 3 healthy meals a day, plus your binge food, or whatever else you think you should

---

* Of course, it is understood that you will avoid foods that you know you are allergic to or have a known physical reaction to—use common sense.

do. You will have time for all of that healthy stuff after this problem is addressed. But I strongly recommend you take a daily multivitamin with minerals.

I have to add a comment here that I am recommending this solution from my own personal experience, not as a representative of any health organization. This is the only strategy that totally cleared me of all binging behavior.

Q.

The Comfort Connection Method in this book seems like it might work to help me in other areas of my life. Is this possible?

A.

Absolutely! I actually developed this method in order to help me perform music in front of audiences with more joy and composure. I had such great success, that I literally apply the techniques to all of my challenges. You can do this also—just change the wording and mental pictures as needed.

We are often unable to see

the endless blue sky

because we are too busy

looking down at our feet.

(PAS)

CHAPTER NINE

STUDY GUIDES

STEP ONE

Describe five things about which you have been feeling guilty regarding your eating, fitness or weight. After each description, write a phrase which will help you lose this guilt. (For example, "I will not criticize myself for eating cookies today.")

1.)

2.)

3.)

4.)

5.)

STEP TWO

List five comfort pay-offs for the over-weight you, and how you can picture living without each:

1.)

Pamela Aye Simon, M.S, R.D., L.D

2.)

3.)

4.)

5.)

STEP TWO continued

List and describe in detail five soothing pay-offs

for the new, thinner you:

1.)

2.)

3.)

4.)

5.)

STEP THREE:

Imagine five scenarios with you as a thinner person.

Take your time with this one. Close your eyes if possible. Let your imagination soar! Describe every detail of each situation.

Picture yourself actually inside the situations, as a person who feels fit and confident, a person who is an example of permanent weight loss. Who are you with? Where are you (describe the setting)? What are you thinking? What are you feeling? What are you wearing? Make these situations similar to those you encounter now, but imagine that you are thinner in these pictures.

1.)

2.)

Pamela Aye Simon, M.S, R.D., L.D

3.)

4.)

Pamela Aye Simon, M.S, R.D., L.D

5.)

CHAPTER TEN

MY MISSION

It is my belief (as both a health professional and a

person

who is struggling to stay fit!), that diet and

exercise changes alone do not succeed in helping

people attain

stable weight management and enhanced fitness

levels.

This is because the changes have not

reached deeply enough. And one more diet, pill, or

exercise plan

won't yield different results.

We need to implement change at the foundational

level of body

image. Every person has a pre-existing mental

picture of what

they look like at their present weight, and what

they think

they should look like

They may also have a belief that they will look

like the other out-of-shape people in their family,

no matter how

hard they try.

This mental picture carries with it lots of guilt for the

discrepancy between the past (or ideal weight) and present. No

matter how much their body then changes for the better with a

new diet and/or exercise program, within 2 years, old behaviors

will unconsciously reappear. The old mental body image (i.e. mental

picture of the out of shape person) will automatically become

reality once again. It is most comfortable in this familiar reality.

Self esteem drops & guilt increases.

Once again, serious attempts at fitness serve only

to increase

negative body confidence and image.

But we can replace that mental image! That mental

picture can

be changed in a completely positive way. And this is

the

foundational work everyone must do to allow for

permanent

change. Positive body imaging is a science. It works

because it

helps change an individual for the better at a

deeper level.

Pamela Aye Simon, M.S, R.D., L.D

PRETEND

It had been such a long day...

with kids and pets to care for

and messes to clean up...

I almost missed it...

I didn't really expect an answer

when I casually asked my young child,

What is the meaning of the word...PRETEND?"

One word is all she said...

BELIEVE

NOTES

Pamela Aye Simon, M.S, R.D., L.D

<u>NOTES</u>

<u>NOTES</u>

Pamela Aye Simon, M.S, R.D., L.D

<u>NOTES</u>

<u>NOTES</u>

<u>NOTES</u>

<u>NOTES</u>

Pamela Aye Simon, M.S, R.D., L.D

<u>NOTES</u>

ABOUT THE AUTHOR

Pamela Aye Simon is a registered, licensed dietitian in private practice in Illinois. She received her Bachelor of Science Degree from Indiana University of Pennsylvania, and earned her Master of Science Degree in Clinical Nutrition from Rush University in Chicago, Illinois. Since then, Ms. Aye Simon has been active in the area of nutrition research and weight control.

From her positions as a research dietitian implementing dietary counseling for clinical trials, to study manager in charge of monitoring the operations of a feeding study, her experiences have allowed her a unique prospective on the weight loss dilemma.

In addition, her private practice and her own personal journey through the world of programs for weight control make this author an excellent resource for others who struggle or work with the weight loss process.

Ms. Aye Simon has co-authored numerous research articles, which have been published in scientific journals.

This is her first book.

Pam Aye Simon welcomes your comments. For all communications, including lecture or workshop requests, contact her at : psimon36@aol.com.

www.ingramcontent.com/pod-product-compliance
Lightning Source LLC
Chambersburg PA
CBHW051447280526
45785CB00003B/1467